MEN|

VERTIGO
VERTIGO

**ABOUT VERTIGO
ABOUT DIZZINESS
AND WHAT YOU CAN DO
ABOUT IT**

VERTIGO
VERTIGO

Copyright©2012 by Meniere Man

All rights reserved. No reproduction, copy or transmission of this Publication may be made without written permission from the author. No paragraph of this publication may be reproduced, copied or transmitted. Save with written permission or in accordance with provisions of the Copyright, Designs and Patents Act 1988, or under the terms of any license permitting limited copying, issued by the Copyright Licensing Agency, The Author has asserted his right to be identified as the author of this work in accordance with the Copyright, Design and Patents Act 1988

Vertigo Vertigo. About Vertigo. About Dizziness And What You Can Do About it. ISBN 978-0-9807155- 2-1 is published by Page Addie, Australia, Page Addie, Australia is an imprint of Page-Addie Press , Great Britain. Vertigo Vertigo is the second edition. First edition published as Meniere Man And The Movie Director ISBN 978-0-9556509- 9-4 BIC Subject category: VFJB A catalogue record for this book is available from the British Library. 1. vertigo 2. dizziness. 3. dizzy. 4. meniere's disease. 5 meniere 6. inner ear. 7. disease symptoms. 8 vestibular problems. 9. vertigo symptoms. 10 causes of vertigo. 11. imbalance in ear. 12. what is vertigo. 13 low salt. 14 coping with vertigo.

Disclaimer: The opinions in this book are strictly the Author's and in no way are meant to take the place of advice by medical professionals. This book is merely written to assist with information as experienced by the Author

Contents

Meniere Man And The Movie Director
7
How Long Does A Vertigo Attack Last?
9
The Mechanics Of A Vertigo Attack
11
Vertigo vs Dizziness
17
The Vertigo And I
21
Meniere's Syndrome
27
Predicting Vertigo
29
The Story Of Vertigo
31
How To Manage The Beginning Stage
Of A Meniere's Attack.
35
How To Manage The Middle Stage
Of A Vertigo Attack
41
How To Manage The End Stage
Of A Vertigo Attack
47
Breath Of Life
55
Getting Through Vertigo
59
Hands For First Aid
61

Pharmacy Rescue
63

Triggers
67

A Change For The Better
69

The Fat Wallet
71

The Ups And Downs
72

A Balanced Meniere's Diet
73

Salty Talk
77

Primo Potassium
85

Fast Fat Food
89

The Unloving Spoon Full
91

The Source Of Good Carbs
93

Balance Rehabilitation
95

Cawthorn-Cooksey Vestibular Exercises
103

Vertigo Training In The Gym
107

Identity
109

Feeling Bad Can Be Good
111

About Meniere Man
115

Meniere Man And The Movie Director

Alfred Hitchcock, a movie director well-known for stranding his characters on the edge of a cataclysm, made a famous psychological thriller called Vertigo in 1958. The term vertigo was and often is incorrectly used to describe a fear of heights. Acrophobia is the name for the dizzy feeling that's often experienced when looking down from a high place.

Real vertigo in Meniere's, is the sensation of horizontal or rotational spinning, which can last between 30 minutes to an hour or for many hours. Spontaneous vertigo can happen at any time. The unpredictable nature of meniere attacks is the reason why you feel constantly on the edge of the vertigo cataclysm. It's not a psychological thriller. It's a reality horror story that everyone diagnosed with meniere's experiences. Vertigo is one of the more dynamic and frightening symptoms of Meniere's disease.

Many Meniere's sufferers are driven to radical surgery in order to get relief from vertigo. However, I found that personal management techniques made it possible for me to cope with vertigo. Now I'm vertigo free. I weight train, windsurf, surf, snowboard, climb ladders and mountains and do balancing core work on a Swiss ball. I started in the early stages of Meniere's disease. Now I have a balanced life. Not bad for a guy who at one time had serious trouble bending over to pick up a ball to throw to his daughter.

In the following chapters, I'll share my techniques and experiential knowledge to help you find your own management system for vertigo.

How Long Does A Vertigo Attack Last?

Everyone is different and no vertigo experience is exactly the same. Vertigo attacks also vary in intensity and duration. You may have a sudden attack that lasts for an eternity of 30 minutes. At other times, you may have signals that a vertigo attack is about to happen…but it doesn't. At other times you may feel 'woozy' for weeks between 'major' vertigo attacks. Other times, you may experience one vertigo attack after another. Or go for days, week, even months without having a vertigo attack. But once a vertigo attack starts, it's anyone's guess as to how long the particular episode will last. Acutely distressing bouts of vertigo can last minutes to hours. Some even lasts for eight or more hours.

The unpredictable nature of the attacks, make the unknown duration and intensity of each episode even more frightening. As human beings we need to know what is going on. The unknown terrifies us. The good news is you can take control of vertigo. With breathing techniques, exercise, diet, medication, meditation and supplements, you can cope better. In time, it's possible to avoid the seemingly inevitable attacks of vertigo.

The Mechanics Of A Vertigo Attack

The most unpredictable and frightening symptom of Meniere's disease is vertigo. The vertigo in Meniere's disease is thought to result from an accumulation of excessive fluid in parts of the inner ear finally resulting in a rupture of membranes which sees a mixing of different fluids; mainly the perilymph and the endolymph. The result is a vertigo attack.

In order to better understand Meniere's disease and vertigo, it is important to have a basic knowledge of the structure and function of the inner ear. The inner ear is a delicate membranous sense organ encased in an hard bony shell. The inner ear is suspended in a fluid known as perilymph. The main composition of which is sodium salts. Inside the membranous inner ear, another fluid circulates. This fluid is called endolymph. Its main composition is potassium.

Inside the membranous inner ear are two chambers called the scalae media and scalae vestibule. Only the scalae media contains endolymph, (potassium) while the scalae vestibule only contains perilymph (sodium). The scalae media and the scalae vestibule are separated by a membrane, called the reissner's membrane. The reissner's membrane's primary function is to act as a diffusion barrier, allowing nutrients to travel from the perilymph to the endolymph chambers.

The inner ear system is complicated, intricate and delicate. The inner ear has it's own immune function which means that the body recognized the ultimate importance of maintaining a separate healthy organ of balance, in order to survive. Without it, as you know, normal function is impossible. Sometimes, as is the case in Meniere's disease, things get tricky.

No one knows for sure what happens. But it is thought, fluid pressure builds up and stretches the reissner membrane that divides the two scalae compartments. As the membrane stretches, the symptoms of a vertigo attack start to happen. It's in this 'infancy' of an oncoming attack, you'll experience your hearing and tinnitus getting worse. But the worst is yet to come. As the membrane becomes severely stretched, the fluids of the inner ear may rupture the reissner. This results in the mixing of the scalae fluids, one rich in sodium, and the other rich in potassium. These fluids mix and flood the vestibular. It's this mixing and flooding that brings on the vertigo. After the membranes rupture, they immediately start to repair and heal, that's when you feel the vertigo diminishing.

Unfortunately with every attack, some hearing is usually permanently lost. This hearing loss happens because the small hairs that help transport sound to the nerve of hearing are damaged in the flood and unfortunately, these do not repair. The more vertigo attacks you have, the more permanent hearing loss.

The functions of the vestibular system

are to sense angular acceleration, linear acceleration (the physics of body motion) and to coordinate head and eye movements as well as maintain the antigravity and lower body muscles in relation to the head. The semicircular canals provide sensation for angular acceleration. So any disturbance of the system has serious consequences for your balance.

Knowing all of this provides you with an intellectual understanding of the mechanics of what is going on when you are having a vertigo attack. The more you know, the more you can self-help your condition.

Here's one example of how understanding the working structure of your inner ear can be helpful. During the attacks one is helpless and as the attack subsides one is still helpless. But as I was lying still trying to get my vertigo under control I began to use a visualization technique that I found helpful. It gave me a sense of positive self healing. I felt as though I was helping in my own recovery, rather than waiting for it to be over. I used the knowledge of the inner ear structure, especially the reissner membranes and scalae fluids. I visualized a healing of the reissner membrane. Then the fluids passing naturally through the reissner. Then an even flow of life fluids in my inner ear. Next, my inner ear slowly returning to a natural, but stable balanced state. I did this repeatedly, during the later stages of the attack, until I was comfortable. Each time I did this I told my self I was healing and getting stronger and that balance was a natural state. Try it and see how it works for you. Accept that balance is a natural body state. Believe it as you do it.

Vertigo vs Dizziness

We talk about vertigo. We talk about dizziness. But what exactly is the difference between dizziness and Meniere's vertigo? Is vertigo just a more intensive form of dizziness? All vertigo comes with dizziness, but not all dizziness comes with vertigo. In most cases of dizziness, dizziness is not vertigo.

Vertigo is a lot different to feeling light headed and dizzy. Vertigo is an overwhelming sensation that the room is spinning around you. So even though you are lying or sitting still, the room feels to you, like it is moving around your body at an incredible speed. But of course it's an illusion.

The room is the room; your kitchen, the living room, a hotel room, a restaurant, or the interior of a plane. The room you are spinning in, is just a 'room'. In reality a room is a noun for an area within a building or structure, enclosed by a floor, a ceiling, and walls. But your reality with vertigo has done an alarming shift. For you, the whole room is spinning. It is no longer the concrete noun. And it becomes much worse when you move your head even a millimeter. Your brain is in alarm mode and with extra body movement it now receives extra signals that you are moving as well and this complicates the already mixed signals it's getting. So don't move. Or let anyone else move you. Tell this to people in your family so when you are having an attack they understand.

This massive equilibrium issue feels as if you are at sea in a hurricane; enough to make you vomit and become terrified. This violent out of control nature of things is what makes Meniere's frightening. So with Meniere's vertigo, you are often 'spinning out' and have your head in a bowl vomiting at the same time. Not a pretty sight.

If someone walks into the room while you are 'spinning out' they will have no understanding of the inner spin you are involved with. They don't see or experience anything different. They are 'normal' but you are in a roller coaster and it's no funfair either. It's hard for anyone to contemplate what you are feeling right at that moment. You are alone in your distressing nightmare. This dynamic illusion of movement makes vertigo different from plain dizzy or common dizziness.

The Vertigo And I

If you have Meniere's disease, unfortunately you'll have a history which involves episodes of true whirling vertigo. It's impossible to forget the experience of a horizontal spinning vertigo attack.

If you're anything like me, the first vertigo attack is the one you remember in detail. You were not aware of the pattern leading up to it. The attack would have sent you and your family rushing off to see the family doctor. You had no idea what was happening to you. This severe vertigo was way beyond dizzy, or the feeling you get when you've drunk a little too much alcohol. Words like dreadful, awful, terrible never match what you're feeling during an attack. Meniere's vertigo symptoms defy description.

You most probably turned up at the Doctor's surgery gripping hold of your friend's arm. The doctor would have noted: showing significant physical and mental distress, looked pale and sweaty. On medical examination vital signs show elevated blood pressure, rapid pulse, nystagmus. Patient breathing faster than normal. All you would have been thinking is, quick, give me a shot of something to make it stop! Well that's all I thought with my first attack. If you were lucky the doctor would have given you an injection of stemetil and the symptoms would have subsided and you were back home sleeping. Oh the heaven of escaping that hellish place of vertigo.

Later your doctor would have arranged for you to see an Otolaryngologist. After hearing tests and historical information about dizziness and vertigo, *my* Specialist sat me down, cleared his throat and took a deep breath, and said, "You've got Meniere's disease. It is an extremely aggressive condition and medical science knows little about".

I ask the question. "What is that?" He went on to explain: Fluctuating hearing loss (sometimes good or bad). Episodic vertigo (can be violent). Tinnitus or ringing in the ears (usually low tone roaring) and Aural fullness (pressure, discomfort). And it's incurable." Severe shock! An incurable disease. Definitely the worst moment in my life. People had labelled me with a few names before. Incorrigible, yes. But never incurable.

Always the optimist, I still asked the question. "Can I recover from this?" And got the following answer. "As I have said before, it is incurable, but the outcome is variable, since the disease pattern of exacerbation and remission makes evaluation of treatment and prognosis difficult to predict. My best advice right now is to go home and rest. Cut down on salt and keep away from stress. And here's a prescription for stemetil and betahistine."

Keep away from stress? Not possible! I was very stressed out. Still the eternal optimist, I asked, "I have organized a family skiing trip, do you think I should go? "Sure, life is short. Go out and enjoy yourself." His last remark puzzled more than anything he had told me! Maybe it was the way he said it? That was about it. Stand up. Walk out the door.

Well, I did go to the mountain the following weekend, with a medical stamp of approval. And the sky was blue. The powder was fresh. And Meniere's was left behind or so I thought. I was a newbie at this point. But on the way home we had to stop the car, change drivers and I lay on the back seat with the kids, for the six hour winding mountain road trip home in the dark. I was now getting the idea about Meniere's. Although on this occasion the timing wasn't all bad. That trip back from the mountain made me realize that with Meniere's disease, I could still do life. For me getting out there when I could, became part of the cure for this incurable optimist.

A month later a friend was flying over from Canada to go fishing with me. Again something organized before the diagnosis. Rather than cancelling him out, I continued with the plans. The plan was to go sea fishing and then travel by car to remote rivers and go fly fishing in the wilderness for a week.

I did wonder if I was capable of going on such an adventure. But sometimes all it takes is a new focus and the support of a good friend. You end up doing far more than you imagine you can. Rather than having a calendar of cancelled plans and empty days. It's about taking a positive approach to living life. I recommend you don't waste a moment waiting for Meniere's to go away. Live as much as you can. Live with Meniere's. Live despite the diagnosis. It's not going away in the short term.

Meniere's disease tends to 'burn out' over time. Some say seven years. Others of course have had it longer than this and it has become a life long condition. But you don't have to wait. You can predict and reduce the number of vertigo attacks, decrease the duration and intensity, recover your equilibrium quickly and live a full and active life; between the time when you are diagnosed with Meniere's and until the time of burnout.

I recovered an active life long before the classic burnout theory. Sure, I was still suffering Meniere's vertigo attack. And I was really worried about how my hearing was progressively deteriorating in my left ear. And how my tinnitus was increasing in volume. But despite these facts, by using the patterns that I had recognized, I worked with my Meniere's and took every opportunity to get out there and do life.

I even surprised my insurance company, or should I say their detectives. They quickly decided that I was far too active and cancelled my Income Continuance Insurance Policy. Apart from that financial disaster, I am proof that working towards getting better as soon as you can, using personal management techniques, will enhance your daily life.

What I figured out is this; you simply can't afford to wait until you feel better. You must start to move in the direction of wellness. There are many ways I did this. From changing my diet, to reducing stress, to doing more exercise, practicing meditation, taking medication, supplements and applying cognitive thinking techniques.

Talking about Meniere's vertigo and what you can do to help yourself, recover a full and active life is what this book is all about. If I can do it, so can you.

Meniere's Syndrome

Meniere's is commonly described as a syndrome combining vertigo, fluctuating low frequency hearing loss, tinnitus and an aural pressure sensation. The symptoms may not necessarily occur simultaneously. Meniere's causes severe disabling and distressing unpredictable vertigo. The sudden episodes of vertigo arrive spontaneously.

Coping With Vertigo

When you have been diagnosed with Meniere's disease, fact is, you are going to have attacks of vertigo. How you cope is a personal choice. Some people cope in ways that others would not contemplate. Vincent Van Gogh, the Impressionist painter placed himself in and out of institutions and struggled to a point of causing himself physical damage, by removing the offending ear! The author Jonathan Swift wrote a book about a giant of a man who travelled through an unknown land, in Gulliver's Travels; the man was, at some point in the story, tied down to the ground and unable to move. Jonathan Swift was a sufferer of Meniere's disease. Peggy Lee, the singer, was another sufferer and she sang soul moving Blues. Alan Shepard the astronaut had surgical intervention. Meniere Man managed Meniere's vertigo, by taking prescribed medication while taking an alternative holistic self help management approach in order minimize and eliminate vertigo.

I believe I made a positive out of a negative. I used Meniere's as a motivation to change my life and live a healthy active life. It has worked. I feel great!

Predicting Vertigo

Vertigo attacks are the most relentless and violent in the early stages of Meniere's disease. Vertigo attacks come at you with a vengeance. One month of Meniere's vertigo, feels like all the worst times of your life slammed together. You spend days in bed or lying on the floor in the bathroom. After an acute attack, you feel exhausted and unsteady, for hours to days. Your life is in disarray. It's literally a tornado ripping through your life.

The timing and frequency of attacks is unpredictable; which creates numerous insecurities and an overall lack of confidence.

You feel vulnerable, uncertain, and lack confidence, possibly for the first time in your life. Meniere's doesn't even fit into a convenient parcel of... I'm not well at the moment but I'll be back in a day or two, when I'm better. Attacks can take on a completely random patterns and can happen anytime, anyplace. It's a very disruptive condition. But over time, after I had experienced a lot of attacks, I was able to read the signals and regularly predict an attack. Once you are able to crystal ball what's happening, you begin to feel a modicum of control. This gives you a sense of 'normality' returning to your life.

You soon come to understand that there are elements to the Meniere's vertigo attack that don't involve spinning. You may have noticed leading up to the vertigo attack, specific sensations that usually warn you an attack is about to happen. These are: sense of ear fullness developing, decreased hearing, feeling of instability and a disturbing increase in roaring tinnitus. If you haven't noticed, *take note* because it can really help you. It is so constructive to be aware of all the elements in an attack.

The Story Of Vertigo

I could see that a Meniere's vertigo attack had a build up, beginning, middle and an end. That B.M.E pattern, Beginning, Middle and End is like a story, or a life journey. Most things in nature have recognizable patterns. When we recognize patterns we lose the chaos and start to find understanding. The recognition that my Meniere's had a pattern, was a major step forward physically and psychologically for me.

When you understand the mechanics

of an attack, as I've described in the previous chapter on Mechanics of Vertigo. You can see a correlation between the B.M.E pattern of the attack. And the physiological changes happening in your ear. What is physiologically going on inside your inner ear, is reflected in how the symptoms feel. Knowing this, gave me a sense of control and predictability, where previously there was only a frightening chaotic Meniere's condition.

Why is finding a pattern to the chaos so important? The mind seeks patterns which we then find meaning in. Something with a pattern becomes familiar. And understandable, like a trip to the mountain, a birth of a new baby, or green leaves emerging in Spring. While Meniere's is not something you look forward it also has a pattern you can recognize. So, if you look at the attacks like a pattern, you can hopefully make sense of these and see the nature in them.When you see the pattern, you can start to look at how to work with the attacks. Then integrate Meniere's into your social life, friends, family, work and holiday times. Another part of the pattern is the period between episodes. There were times when I'd feel completely symptom free except for the continual tinnitus. During these times I did as much as was sensible. These times were like gifts of near normality where life was life as I knew it. Laws of gravity seemed to apply.

So how do you recognize that a vertigo attack is on its way? You can't always tell, especially if you are busy and 'push' any approaching symptoms aside. But if you are aware of the stages, you are in a better position to manage the situation. Becoming conscious of stages takes practice.

The way I see it, there are three stages of Meniere's Vertigo. The time just prior to a Vertigo attack, Beginning; during a vertigo attack, Middle; and the time as the attack is ending, End. I call it the B.M.E. Beginning, Middle and End. Once you understand there are three stages to the attacks, B.M.E. you can apply coping techniques and smart management to each specific stage. That is how I felt I gained control over a disease that was controlling me. When you are able to take responsibility through knowledge, you can really make improvements to your health. Physically, mentally and emotionally.

How To Manage The Beginning Stage Of A Meniere's Attack.

In the first stage, if you're observant, you'll notice increased tinnitus. This signals two things. Firstly you are overdoing things or you have drunk or eaten the wrong things. Tinnitus will be your first signal that you are getting into the zone for an attack. Also an aural fullness, the feeling of cotton wool packed into the ear which is making hearing more difficult and the fullness feels uncomfortable. This is where the reissner membrane is being stretched and fluid is building up in your vestibular. You may also find yourself off balance. All of these symptoms may take place over a day or so. This is the first stage leading up to a vertigo attack. Or the Beginning.

There are many simple ways to cope in the beginning stages of an attack. The sooner you recognize the symptoms of this beginning stage the better. If you take action at this stage you'll have more chance of avoiding the attack. Or lessening the intensity.

When the symptoms of increased tinnitus, fullness in your ear, hearing difficulty and unsteadiness appear, stop doing what you're doing immediately. Or at least within the next 20 minutes. Don't keep at what your doing for any longer than 20 minutes. Lie down or put your feet up and relax. Practice deep breathing exercises. The more oxygen you can get into your body, the better. Don't watch T.V. or work on the computer. Rest your eyes. Remember the eyes, are directly connected to your vestibular system. Don't drive.

If you are experiencing beginning symptoms of a Meniere's vertigo attack, you need to put measures in place for a day or two. I'm serious. This is the time to pay attention to your body and take more care in certain areas.

Pay attention to known triggers of attacks. Don't drink alcohol or artificial drinks that contain sugars. Say no to your wake-up cup of coffee. Certain teas like chamomile, raspberry, rose hip or peppermint are soothing. You must find something palatable to substitute for caffeine. You can sweeten herbal teas with honey. Or make your own tea by mixing 1 teaspoon fresh grated ginger root and 1 teaspoon honey in a cup of boiling water. Drink as needed. Hot lemon and honey makes a great drink too. Lemon is now being discussed as a possible help for vertigo symptoms.

Eat small protein-rich meals. (This causes less hyperactivity in the stomach, according to a study done at Penn State University). Don't eat salted foods. I also find a banana, which is rich in potassium, seems to settle things down.

Ginger oil in a carrier oil such as almond oil, massaged gently on the stomach helps with nausea. Take a hot bath or a shower with a few drops of essential oils added to help relaxation, like lavender. I would lay in the bath, filling and refilling with hot water, until the taps ran cold. Baths really helped me relax and stop feeling of anxiety and panic.

You can practice relaxation methods you've learned. This relaxation and cessation of activities is not just for half an hour. It's for as long as it takes until symptoms go away. Do everything you can to relax, eat and drink, avoid triggers. If you don't know how to relax effectively or eat the right foods and avoid trigger foods. You may need to read up and do some research. This will help you to determine what works best for you.

I found that by treating this beginning stage seriously, I managed to avoid some of the vertigo attacks all together. This was also because I had changed aspects of my life style towards taking more care of diet, stress and physical exercise as well.

I have written a comprehensive book called '*Let's Get Better: A Memoir of Meniere's disease*', which covers these areas in more detail. But of course you may have found, or being doing other activities that work for you.

Whatever you do, take this beginning stage seriously. And give yourself a good chance of of avoiding attacks of vertigo.

How To Manage The Middle Stage Of A Vertigo Attack

The second stage. vertigo is the most dynamic stage of the Meniere's attack. At this stage you may have only a few minutes to realize that there is no going back. You'll definitely be experiencing serious dizziness which is quickly developing into nystagmus, where your eyes feel like they're following the room moving around you. This may take place over three to four minutes, but you are still mobile enough to find a place to lie down. After that, you are into a rotational spinning vertigo attack. This lasts for at least 30 minutes to an hour. Towards the end of the attack you will notice the spinning is a little less severe. As the spinning slows down, you are managing to see something specific in the room before it then spins away. Slowly you are able to focus on a window or a picture. Once focusing on an object becomes possible, you start feeling you can get control back. It helps to stay focused on one spot for another 30 minutes or so. Finally, there is no more spinning and you may be able to sleep.

You have read in the mechanics of a vertigo attack that it follows a physiological pattern. Like most medical events, a fever, a wound healing…Meniere's vertigo follows a pattern too. That means once the attack starts, you know there will be specific phases to the attack. Then the attack will finish. It's a pattern, like any natural phenomenon. The way blood is pumped through the heart; the way contractions are a pattern of birth. The sun rising and sinking. Think of Meniere's as having a natural pattern of activity, and accept the pattern as it is happening. Knowing it will complete its natural cycle.

As soon as you notice the symptoms described in the beginning stages of vertigo, you must take steps and act. Sounds obvious, but unless you do, you won't have any warning and suddenly you'll find yourself in an acute spinning attack. You may be on the street in a meeting or having dinner with friends. Not the best place to lay prostrate vomiting.

When the attack begins, lay down. Make yourself as comfortable as possible. Turn down the lights. Avoid noise. A quiet room helps you relax more. The more you can relax, the less severe your symptoms will be. And the sooner you will recover your equilibrium.

Don't lie down flat. Place two or more pillows under your head. Don't shut your eyes completely. Leave them slightly open. And softly out of focus. Don't try to use your eyes to keep track of the furniture moving around the room. Or stop the spinning. You will only feel worse and become more anxious.

During an attack, listen to your interior voice. Change negative self talk into positive self talk. Your mind is something that you can control. Interrupt yourself and stop any negative thoughts you having. Negative self talk increases anxiety. Stop yourself and change each negative thought for a positive one. Use encouraging words like "I am O.K. It will pass." "It's just another Meniere's attack." Talk it down in importance.

The more you minimize the cycle of anxiety, the less fear you have. Mind over matter works well for Meniere's. Remind yourself that you are not in any danger and the Meniere's attack will pass. The attack you are experiencing is not a permanent state. You won't be trapped in this experience forever. This type of awareness helps reduce anxiety and stress.

As the spinning subsides a little try to find a focus on something, just above eye level directly in front of you. A picture, a spot on the wall, or a door handle. Whatever is in front of you. You may not be able to focus this way, until the attack lessens. But do it as soon as you can. If the spot slides away slowly bring your focus back to the point. Repeat this until it is possible to stay focused on that point. At this stage you know that the reissner is healing and you will soon be in the recovery stage.

Avoid any movements. When you move

your head, even a millimeter. The vestibular nerve is already challenged with the attack. So any other demands only intensify the sense of feeling unsteady and flying off into another spinning. If you have to change position, change *very, very slowly.*

At this point you may be able to do a healing visualization. I visualized the reissner's membrane healing and the balancing fluids passing naturally through the reissner membrane. Finaly I visualized the calm waters of a lake. And my whole being stable, calm and balanced. I did this repeatedly, during the later stages of the attack, until I was comfortable. Each time I did this I told my self I was healing and getting stronger and that balance was a natural state.

Next time you are experiencing a vertigo attack, tell yourself; the cycle has begun; now I'm moving forwards and it will come to an end. It's a temporary state. Relax and ride it out, go with it. I don't want to sound glib here, but if you don't fight against it, the spinning seems less intense. And the less shock you have, the quicker your body will naturally repair the situation.

When we catch a cold or flu, we feel awful physically, but we know that we will get better. I know the symptoms of a Meniere's attack are far worse than a common cold, but the principle is the same. You must tell yourself, convince yourself that the attacks always pass.

Remember, the more you relax and go with it, the quicker the vertigo will appear to resolve. The more you panic, the more anxious you get, the worse the symptoms appear and the longer it seems to go on. So the real trick in coping at this stage is this. Use your mind control and don't fight against it. Relax as deeply as you can.

Ironically, the more vertigo you experience, the easier it gets to know the pattern of it. You become less anxious and the attacks don't seem as bad.

Becoming aware of the pattern, is about gaining a sense of control. This kind of awareness is key to making a huge difference in the severity of the attack. Detaching the mind from the experience allows the experience to be what it is. Work on controlling fear and anxiety.

How To Manage The End Stage Of A Vertigo Attack

Well it's more of a recovery stage. Emotionally you feel a great sense of relief. During this final stage, the vertigo has stopped and you have slept or rested for a couple of hours. You may even be able to get up at this point; or stay right where you are. You will find yourself wondering exactly what can I do without going back into an attack. The feeling in this stage is one of vulnerability. You are no dizzy but not stable either. I call it woozy.

You can't be physically decisive at this stage. Balance is not fully restored. But you're pleased to be back in the land of gravity once again. Where chairs and walls don't move around the room. And the only things still moving are the hands on the clock.

It takes time to gain a sense of full recovery from an attack. I found after the attack I was in a recovery mode for a few days. This stage is a physiological healing time. If you try to push through this end stage you may undo the healing that is taking place. And find yourself back having another attack. At this point, you can feel woozy and you should walk slowly. You won't be able to concentrate or do physically demanding activities. You'll be feeling very tired and will need to rest regularly.

This end stage can take from 3 days to a week. Although this is more of a personal time frame. This is a very valuable time for healing. And you must take advantage to heal well. It does take time. Learn to listen to your body. If you have suffered a severe vertigo episode that has left you exhausted. Listen to your common sense telling you to rest and sleep. Remember you are in a recovery mode and need to replenish and heal your body. An attack is a serious physiological trauma. When you've recovered you can get going and get active.

Drink and Recover

Drink water. Hydrate yourself to counter the effects of body shock. Stay hydrated after a vertigo attack. Drink water with high levels of magnesium and low sodium content. Avoid caffeine. Or caffeinated drinks. Caffeine increases dehydration. And that's not what you need at this stage.

When you can get up and make yourself a drink, then even the small action of grating ginger root to make yourself warm tea, is personally empowering. Small actions go a long way to recovery. Try a cup of ginger tea. This can be made by washing and peeling fresh ginger root and grating it into a teapot. One tablespoon of grated ginger makes about four cups. Pour boiling water over. Seep for 5 minutes. Sweeten with a teaspoon or two of unprocessed natural honey. Sip slowly. Drink hot or cold. A word of warning though.

Do not take ginger if you have a bile duct

obstruction or gallstones. Ginger may stimulate bile production. High doses of ginger (6 grams or more) can cause damage to the stomach lining and ulcers. Ginger can cause allergic skin reactions. Consult your doctor before taking ginger if you take blood thinners.

Also green tea is a natural source of antioxidants. Or a large glass of freshly squeezed orange juice. Drink it slowly "chewing" each mouthful so the vitamin C is absorbed through the mucus membranes in your mouth.

Eat and Recover

Eat a banana. Potassium rich, and with natural sugars, a banana gives your body a much needed boost of vitamins, minerals and energy to get you back on your feet quickly. For a quick natural pick up of blood sugar levels. Eat poppy seeds or a few almonds, raisins, figs, apricots, or cranberries.

Use Water to Recover

Take a long hot bath with essential oils to relax your nerves. Or a hot shower. Let the water run over the back of your neck and down your spine. Breathe and relax. Shake your hands as you let go the vertigo experience. The properties of water remove negative ions from your body. This will refresh and relax you.

Use Oil to Recover

100% pure essential oils can calm tensions, relieve stress and help promote restful and repairing sleep. Relaxing lavender, soothing ylang ylang or rose, balancing geranium, or naturally calming mandarin orange.

Place 5-10 drops of oil with warm water into a perfume burner for essential oils. Breathe in the scent in the room and you will feel the stress release. Mix a few drops of your choice of oils into a warm bath.

Mix two drops with a carrier oil such as almond oil for a self massage of your feet. Or have someone who cares for your well-being; give you a gentle whole body massage, especially your shoulders and back.

Connect and Recover

Stand outdoors for a moment. Look at the horizon. Breathe. Listen and look around at nature. This act is grounding and re-orientating. And helps reconnect you to the world.

Move and Recover

Correct adjustment to vestibular imbalance, is a process known as compensation. Vestibular compensation is a process that allows the brain to regain balance control and minimize dizziness symptoms. Getting up and moving around as soon as you can, actively assist to help your brain compensate. So, as soon as you feel remotely back to normal, get up and change your focus and perspective. The objective here is to go slowly but definitely get going. When you have an imbalance between, the right and left vestibular organs, the key component to successful adaptation is a dedicated effort to keep moving, despite the symptoms of dizziness and imbalance.

By moving and doing things, (despite feeling 'woozy') you strengthen the balance system. As you move, you're helping your body and brain regain the ability to process balance information.

Do Recover

Do things you like to do, such as spending time with friends and family. Walking. Eating out. Shopping. Don't let your vertigo keep you at home. Move about. Get your circulation going through out your body. Get your brain to take responsibility for your entire body again. Moving about and helps you heal and recover.

Breath Of Life

One of the greatest aids to relaxation is our breath. You can use your breath for first aid. How you breathe affects how you feel. The breath is a powerful tool. Learning to control your breathing takes practice. Concentrating on your breathing is the first thing you can do when vertigo happens. The idea is to use breath to relax and calm yourself.

Using the breath to relax is used in meditation. Yoga is a fantastic discipline to study and breath is a major part of yoga. Also Tai Chi is a great way to control body and breath. You should seriously be looking at one of these disciplines to incorporate into your daily life.

If you tense your body, shallow-breathe or hold your breath, it makes the vertigo attack seem worse. But if you relax your body and breathe slowly and deeply, you get more oxygen into your body and the panic reaction reduces. Join a Yoga or Thai Chi group or you can practice breathing exercises at home. Breathing from your diaphragm oxygenates your blood and helps you relax. Breathing exercises will reduce anxiety and oxygenate your cells. When your cells have oxygen, the body has a greater chance of returning to a healthy state. Practice these breathing exercises before you have an attack, so breathing correctly is automatic.

To breathe deeply, begin by putting your hand on your abdomen just below the navel. Breathe in, as if you are breathing in through your belly. Make your belly fill with air and feel it expand then move the breath up into your chest and feel it expand. Hold the breath for a few seconds, exhale slowly. Inhale again slowly through your nose and watch your hand move out as your belly expands and then move the breath up and expand your chest.

When you exhale, make sure you expel all your breath by pulling in your diaphragm and expelling all the air from your lower lungs. Repeat several times. This takes a little practice to breathe through your belly and then into your chest. This is the natural way the body breathes. It's what we do in our sleep or when we are unconscious. But when we are conscious we tend to breathe only from the chest and consequently make half breaths.

Getting Through Vertigo

When you feel a vertigo attack is about to begin, do the following relaxation exercise. The following breathing and relaxation exercises, need to have been practiced before an attack, so when an attack is imminent, you can do them automatically.

Using the exercise on the next page will give you a great sense of personal power. You'll be controlling your mind and your body. This will help you get through a Meniere's attack.

Close your eyes slowly.
Breathe easily.
Breathe slowly and deeply.
Imagine you can regulate your heart beat.
As you breathe relax your mind.
Relax the muscles in your jaw.
As you breathe relax your body.
Repeat this cycle.

Hands For First Aid

You can use your hands to simply apply physical pressure to help your body sense where it is. Practice these exercises before you have a vertigo attack so you can decide which one makes you the most comfortable. Then if you are able, instigate one during an attack to help you feel a more comfortable and gain a sense of control.

Hand Cup

Cup your hands over your eyes for five seconds while you breathe deeply. The warmth and darkness are comforting.

Hand Press

Half close your eyes; place your right hand across your forehead. Doing this helps your head orient with the rest of your body. Press your forehead against your hand. Practice another version. Place a hand on each side of your head above your ear. Perform the counter-pressure exercise on each side.

Fingertip Press

Place your fingertips on your forehead. Press your forehead against your fingertips. Try to keep your fingers from being pushed back by your head.

After you have had a few Meniere's attacks. And you understand what helps to lesson the severity of the attacks; you may emotionally start to accept those vertigo moments. And begin to integrate them into your life.

Pharmacy Rescue

Medical treatment of Meniere's disease is tailored to each patient. And this will have been discussed between you and your doctor. But here's some medication information you may like to consider and discuss further with your doctor.

Drugs prescribed for acute vertigo should be used sparingly, as they may impair the vestibular adaptation process. The debate on drug effectiveness for acute vertigo continues. There is a school of thought, that rather than medicate, you would do as well with vestibular adaptation exercises or a vestibular rehabilitation program to help manage symptoms.

If medications are required, a 3-month trial of a diuretic (e.g. Dyazide) is often given. Ask for a potassium sparing diuretic. Typically, vestibular suppressants and anti-nausea medications (e.g. meclizine, Compazine) are prescribed to suppress any vertigo symptoms.

There are various anti-vertigo drugs available that can make you feel better during the initial or severe phases of vertigo. Talk to your doctor about these options.

Vestibular sedatives generally only mask the vertigo by decreasing the brain's response to vestibular input. These drugs are Antivert, Droperidol, Compazine, Valium, Ativan.

Other research on vestibular sedatives such as benzodiazepines, antihistamines or prochlorperazine is based, as I understand it, on experimental laboratory animal research. Clinical observation of these drugs effectiveness is anecdotal. At the time of writing, there are no controlled trials.

Diuretics

Diuretics or diuretic-like medications Dyazide, hydrochlorothiazide, actually decrease the fluid pressure load in the inner ear by increasing sodium excretion. But remember they also strip potassium out of your body. Because of this, you need to make sure your have a diuretic that is potassium sparing. There is no singularly effective pharmacological treatment to get rid of vertigo. Don't you wish! But there are prescribed drugs that can help you through an acute episode of vertigo.

Triggers

Avoiding trigger substances (e.g. caffeine) alone may be sufficient. If you don't know your triggers, look on the internet for suspected triggers to give you an idea of food culprits. Also, keep a notebook of what you think your triggers are. Look for clues. What you eat in relation to attacks and write these coincidences down. Maintaining a reduced salt intake to less than 2 grams of sodium intake per day is thought to help keep the cochlear pressure low. If you have eaten food high in salt preceding an attack, for example, you may see a distinct pattern emerging. Take note of what you are doing. You are looking for patterns to help you understand the relationship between triggers and vertigo attacks.

A Change For The Better

Lifestyle and dietary changes are usually the second step after being prescribed drug program. These lifestyle changes are not insignificant. They are vital to your eventual well being. In fact, I made these lifestyle changes and eventually replaced the prescription drugs I was taking.

Pay attention to what you eat and drink and look at your holistic health status. Instead of just focusing on your disease. Dis-ease is disease within the body, so by considering your body and not just its symptoms, you can go a long way to helping your condition.

By looking at smoking, alcohol consumption, exercise; you can make change in your habits; by looking at the stresses you are under and your workload; you can make changes to your profession. If you take a close look at how you are living your life, you can make significant changes that will ultimately improve your health. And help you manage vertigo symptoms.

How you do things is a personal revelation. No one can say for sure what changes you can make. It's something you need to figure for yourself. But there are basic things everyone knows about. From throwing out the salt shaker and tossing the deep fryer, to putting on your trainers and getting out for a walk; your health is up to you. There are so many simple measures you can do. Improve your health status, and by default, you recover a sense of balance in your world.

The Fat Wallet

Health is the most important factor in your life. Health is the real wealth. Money comes and goes, but good health matters more than the size of your wallet. Aim for a simple, uncomplicated life. Don't forget to give yourself personal time and personal space. Make time each day where you do things for you. Just for you. Treat yourself like a friend. Even buy yourself something nice! It's easy to do so much for others. But what about you! Give yourself time through the day for meditation and inner peace.

The Ups And Downs

Pay attention to how you move. Make your movements controlled and fluid rather than sudden. Avoiding sudden movements with your head or body. Avoid tipping your head back to look up. If you need to bend down to pick up things, do this action slowly. At times, simply sitting or lying in one position is considered as one of the most highly recommended vertigo rehabilitation solutions.

A Balanced Meniere's Diet

Eat right to fuel and fortify your body. You can only eat so much in one day. But how are you eating? What goes in your mouth matters. When you make food choices, you are deciding for your body. No one spoon feeds you. It is up to you to eat the kinds of foods that count, rather than empty calories. Make every mouthful matter and you'll see improvements in your overall health, your skin, nails, hair and eyes. Your body reflects your current nutritional status and your body has its own history, which is made up of how you've treated it in the past. You can affect your body in the future by the choices you make today.

Vitamin C is highly beneficial in dealing with Vertigo as natural vitamin c contains riboflavin's which are good for the general circulation of blood. Citrus fruit like oranges, lemons and other fruit like strawberries should be included in your diet. Add lime or lemon peel in cooking, as both are rich in riboflavin's.

Garlic, chilies and ginger also improve the circulatory issues associated with vertigo.

Eat and buy organic meats, fish and poultry. Avoid farmed fish, caged factory chicken and meat treated with hormones, antibiotics and pesticides.

Don't eat processed chips or cookies for a snack. Think in terms of foods that do your body good. Healthy snacks are yogurt (protein, calcium) fresh fruit (vitamin C), and and unsalted nuts such as almonds or walnuts (essential fatty acids). A favorite of mine is fresh or unsweetened pineapple, low fat low salt cottage cheese and a handful of almonds or a mixture of almonds, linseeds, sunflower seeds ground up and sprinkled on top,. Great sources of enriched vitamins and minerals.

Personally, I'm not a health food nut, as the term goes, but I do appreciate, more than ever these days, the taste of real whole food: raw, fresh and organic. Why eat a candy that is artificially flavored to taste like mango. Real food is really good for you. Full of vitamins and nutrients. Control what you put in your mouth. By eating real and healthy foods, you are working towards a vertigo free life.

Salty Talk

It's agreed by experts, that sodium creates an imbalance in the body's fluids, especially in the inner ear. This can trigger vertigo. So the goal for managing Meniere's vertigo is to reduce the total body fluid volume. Which reduces inner ear fluid volume. And the pressure and rupture in the vestibular.

According to the University of Maryland Medical Centre treatment for Meniere's disease "is directed towards attempts to decrease the fluid pressure in the inner ear by avoiding substances that may trigger or exacerbate fluid pressure build up in the inner ear." Sodium causes fluid retention, so you will need to reduce your salt intake. This is done by aggressive salt-restriction. But we are not talking a total no salt diet. Don't try to eliminate salt altogether; your muscles and nerves need it to function. Fact is, the average western diet consumes just over 3,000 milligrams of sodium each day. You can't live without salt, but you don't need as much salt to live! "The goal is to reduce your daily sodium intake to 1500-2000 milligrams. This involves more than not sprinkling salt on your food. It requires diligence in precisely measuring your sodium intake from all sources by inspecting package labels and kitchen habits."

When planning a low salt diet, you can read books on low-salt diets or consult with a Dietitian or Nutritionist to establish a salt-restricted diet and help keep track of your sodium intake. Cutting down on salt is one good thing, but if you eat enough foods rich in potassium, you may not have to cut back so much on the salt. That's where a registered dietitian can help you with a specific diet plan tailored for you.

According to the University of Maryland

Medical Centre, maintaining a low-salt diet involves restricting sodium intake to between 1,500 to 2,000 milligrams per day. That's what you need to be doing as a Meniere's sufferer. This means cutting out more than just salt in cooking or as a condiment.

Pay attention to the nutritional makeup of everyday foods. Maintain a low salt intake on a daily basis. Avoid adding salt to food while cooking. Throw away the salt shaker. Don't add salt to meals at the table. It doesn't make sense to not put salt into the dish you're cooking but shake it over your plate at the table. Salting your food is not an option. Adding salt may be the first habit you give up.

Make an effort to check out what is in your fridge, pantry and cupboards. Take high salt foods out of the house. You must be a food detective here, for your own well-being. One of the best ways to change a habit is to not buy any salt or salted foods or bring them into the house. Let your family know why they need to read labels too. Whoever is cooking dinner, needs to look at how much salt goes into the recipes and modify. That's how friends and family can get involved rather than inadvertently sabotaging or compromising your aim at reducing salt down.

Most sodium comes in the familiar form of table salt. But other chemical compounds also contain sodium. Even diet drinks, such as diet soda, contain sodium. Some brands of bottled water can have high sodium content especially if carbonated. Gas as the Italians call it. Gas or no gas. Just a few primo changes to food and beverage choices, makes a difference to lowering your daily total of sodium.

Read labels and avoid sodium saccharin (a sugar substitute), disodium phosphate (a preservative), monosodium glutamate and trisodium phosphate.

In this following section you may wish to get a high-lighter, as the list of foods to avoid is impressive. Highlight those foods you are using on a regular basis. Then count up how many and see what changes you can make.

Processed Foods

A general low-salt rule, avoid or limit processed foods that are high in sodium, canned vegetables and soups, spaghetti sauce, vegetable juices and ready-to-eat cereals. Avoid high salt foods like ravioli, salted nuts, potato crisps, broth, bouillon cubes and gravies. Delicious as they are, ham, sausage, bacon, liver, offal are also offenders in salt overload.

Don't Do Dairy

Your only use for cheese should be in a mousetrap. This is the end of the cheese board as you know it. Say goodbye to aged cheddar, and blue vein. Gorgonzola, is out. Avoid hard cheeses and soft cheeses including cheese sauces, cheese spreads, processed cheese, processed cheese, and cheese dips. Don't bring cottage cheese, salted butter and margarine into the house unless they are low-fat.

Bakehouse Blues

The more processed a grain is, the more likely it is to be high in sodium. This list is more than a baker's dozen. Breads and rolls, quick breads, self-rising flour, pancake mix, pizza, biscuits, bread crumb coatings, croutons, salted crackers, pretzels, baking soda, and baking powder.

Vege Villans

Juice your own vegetables. Avoid canned and packet vegetable juices, black and green olives, your favorite dill pickles, sauerkraut, pickled vegetables and relishes, pasta and tomato sauces, bottled salad dressings, regular peanut butter, soy sauce and sauces like BBQ, seasonings like rubs and marinades.

Eating Out Low Salt

Meals which are high sodium can trigger vertigo. So avoid fast foods restaurants. Chicken, fish, burgers. All these restaurants use highly seasoned ingredients in their foods.

Asian foods use msg, salt and soy and chili sauce. Mexican foods are cooked with sauces, and added condiments which are all very high in salt or nitrates. Korean food: the sauces, condiments, pickles are high in salt. Indian food, curry sauces, and condiments are near the top of the salt scale.

Big Tick Low Salt Shopping

Many choices of low salt foods are available in supermarkets, food stores and markets. It's easy to replace high salt foods with low-salt foods. Here's an example. Instead of crackers with a high salt content, choose a brand with the lowest salt content. You still eat foods you love, you just have to change the brands and put low salt packets, cans or cartons into your shopping trolley. Spend a few months paying attention to reading labels and making low salt food choices, and soon you understand the brands and products that are right for your health.

We've talked about foods you should avoid. Here's a list of foods you can eat: Low-fat dairy products such as low-salt cheese, lean organic meat, water-packed tuna, fresh or frozen vegetables, fresh or frozen fruits, whole grain bread, low-salt biscuits and crackers. Whole grain cereals such as oats, enriched cereals like Grape nuts, unsalted popcorn, fresh salads, bottled or packet low sodium salad dressings.

Primo Potassium

Potassium is a major positive ion inside human cells and helps cells with body functions, Contracting your muscles requires potassium. From lifting your eyebrow, to lifting a finger. Your heart is a muscle that contracts too. So get potassium for heart function and also brain function.

Reducing the amount of fluid your body retains helps to regulate the fluid volume and pressure in your inner ear. The goal is to reduce fluid pressure in the body. Your doctor may have prescribed a diuretic which you take as a supplement. A diuretic is a medication to reduce fluid retention.

A low-sodium diet combined with a diuretic is often prescribed to patients with Meniere's disease. Taking a diuretic may help control the severity and frequency of vertigo.

A diuretic helps excrete body fluids from the body. This strips the body of salt which is in the fluids of the body. Diuretics make you visit the bathroom more than you normally would. You pass urine more frequently. But when you go to the toilet more frequently, many positive minerals are excreted such as potassium. Your body can't afford to lose important minerals. When you're on a low-sodium diet, your sodium levels in the body are at a minimum. This combination of low salt and diuretics can cause other health problems.

You don't need much salt to live a healthy life, but if your salt level is under the recommended level for a healthy body, that can be a health hazard. So you have to get the balance right. You need some salt and you also need potassium for health.

Potassium has been linked to the prevention of major medical conditions. Potassium is the great 'reducer'. This mineral helps lower blood pressure; reduce the risk of stroke, reduce the risk of heart disease, reduce the chances of developing kidney stones, and amazingly, potassium reduces the body's sensitivity to salt. This reduction of sensitivity is a good reason to ask your doctor about potassium sparing diuretics.

As well as taking a potassium sparing diuretic, you can counteract potassium depletion naturally, by increasing your potassium in your daily diet. Most people consume only about half of the daily recommended amount of potassium. So what foods contain generous helpings of potassium? One abundant source of potassium is avocado. A whole avocado contains around 1,100 mg. A great reason to make guacamole.

Fruits contain large amounts of potassium. The richest sources are bananas, one medium banana has 422 mg. Half cup of fresh plums provides a 530 mg of potassium. A half cup of dried raisins contains nearly 600 mg of potassium. One medium orange, 237 mg.

A medium potato baked with skin on provides 926 mg of potassium. All the following foods contain high levels of potassium.

Cantaloupe melon, apricots, orange juice, sweet potatoes, green beans, broccoli, green peppers, asparagus, Brussels sprouts turnips, parsnips, tomatoes, soybeans, brown rice and garlic. A chocolate fix is good for you. Cocoa and chocolate are high potassium: An ounce of chocolate has about 120 mg of potassium.

Go nuts. Almonds 200 mg. Brazil nuts 170 mg. Sunflower seeds 200 mg of potassium.

Did you know, some spices have high levels of potassium. Just one tablespoon of parsley gives you 16 mg of potassium. So if you make Middle Eastern salad with a cup of chopped parsley, and four cloves of garlic (at 12 mg of potassium each), you're cooking. One teaspoon of dill seeds 25 mg. Other sources of potassium are celery and cress. Once you understand food values, it's easy to cook without salt while increasing your potassium intake.

Experiment with flavours. Instead of salt for taste, use herbs and spices to replace salt in cooking. These add flavour and taste to dishes.

Fast Fat Food

Cholesterol is a waxy substance that travels through the bloodstream to all the body's cells. While cholesterol has important functions in the body, excessive amounts of cholesterol may adversely affect circulation of blood to the inner ear. To help promote blood viscosity and improve blood supply to the inner ear and brain, it's important to reduce the amount of saturated fats and trans fats you eat. These types of fats are commonly found in meats, oils, fast foods and processed foods.

You can control cholesterol levels in the body by controlling the amount of high cholesterol foods you eat. The first step is to throw the deep fryer away. Avoid all fried foods, (especially deep-fried foods), and grill, bake, poach, instead of frying.

The second step to reducing cholesterol, is to reduce your intake of ice cream, cheese, milk, mayonnaise, eggs, butter, and meats, because all these foods are high in fat.

The Mayo Clinic also published a list of the top five foods that can help lower cholesterol levels in the body. Their list of cholesterol reducing foods include: high soluble fiber foods, like oatmeal, apples, pears, prunes and kidney beans; walnuts and almonds; foods high in omega-3 fatty acids, such as tuna, salmon, sardines, canola oil, olive oil; Foods fortified with plant sterols, such a cholesterol reducing margarine, which are designed to assist with blocking cholesterol absorption.

The Unloving Spoon Full

If you love a teaspoon of sugar in your tea, you need to give it up. Sugars raise blood pressure and blood sugar temporarily. When your blood sugar is high, the blood takes longer to circulate to reach your brain. Simple sugars are 'bad' sugars. Because almost as soon as you eat them, they cause a sudden spike,(sugar high) followed by a sudden drop in blood sugar levels. This sudden spike and drop is thought to be a possible trigger for a Meniere's vertigo attack.

To lower the level of blood sugar in your body, it is important to cut out simple carbohydrates and simple sugars from your diet. Instead, go for complex carbohydrates, which are known to stabilize the body's blood sugar levels. When you eat more complex carbohydrates, it helps your body maintain optimum blood sugar balance.

High Sugar Foods To Avoid

The following foods should be reduced or eliminated from your diet: cartooned concentrated fruit juice, candy, cookies, biscuits, cakes, muffins, donuts, sweets, pastas and breads made with white flour, sugary cereals, white sugar, ice cream, milk chocolate (go for dark chocolate).No jams. No soda drinks.

The Source Of Good Carbs

The opposite of the simple sugar spike, is the slow burning energy of complex carbohydrates. When you replace foods with simple sugars for more complex carbohydrates, you feel the benefits. No sugar rushes with highs and lows and you'll find you're less exhausted.

Whole grain bread, brown rice, legumes like dried beans, pulses and lentils, vegetables, barley, wild rice, soy beans, fruits, nuts and seeds. All of these complex carbohydrates have multiple benefits such as reducing cholesterol and giving you more energy. Not only do they taste great, they're a great way to get minerals and vitamins your body needs to heal.

Balance Rehabilitation

If you experience problems with your balance between episodes of vertigo, you may benefit from vestibular rehabilitation therapy to help the development of vestibular compensation. Then you'll be up and about doing the things you want to be doing. Vestibular exercises were not around when I was diagnosed with Meniere's disease, but I have included this updated information in this edition.

No one told me about vestibular rehabilitation, because no one knew. But left to my own to figure this, I went on my 'gut' feeling and decided to do balance sports. I learned balance sports and by doing these sports, my vestibular system would have been compensating. The list is a long one. I walked until I was able to jog; learned to windsurf, learned to wake board, water skied, learned to ski, learned to cross country ski, learned to do weight training, learned how to stretch and do core balance workouts on the Swiss ball, rowed with a rowing machine, cycled, snow boarded, swam in the pool, swam in the ocean, surfed again, climbed ladders, gardened, pruned trees, dug in the garden, read books, worked on the computer, played ball, went sailing, went fishing, snorkelling, traveled by air, by car etc! Phew! I did all of this with attacks of vertigo. I just had to pick my moments. Looking back at moments, like the skiing trip straight after I was diagnosed with Meniere's. The one the doctor ordered.

The six hour drive down to the mountain was along winding roads; at night. Once on the mountain, I climbed up and down snowy and slippery slopes; I skied down hill, went up in a chair lift. I exercised for two days; and then on the drive back home, after the fully active weekend, I had a vertigo attack. No wonder! My balance system spent all weekend doing a full range of compensating tasks. But I think it was well worth the result. Yes I had an attack but I spent normal family time on holiday and enjoyed the great outdoors.

Everything you do helps, whether you snow ski, throw a tennis ball to the dog or plant bulbs in the garden. Every movement incorporates body balance. That's why, when you do things, you can sometimes feel bad. But if you accept dizziness or vertigo as a necessary part of the healing process, fear of doing things won't come into the equation.

When you see dizziness and even a vertigo attack as a sign that an imbalance in your vestibular systems still exists, you need to believe that every physical activity you do, is helping you recover your life. It is like tough love for vertigo. Laying around in bed doesn't help you get anywhere. But getting up and having a go, goes a long way, towards getting a full and active life back again.

See every movement and exercise, whether it is with a physiotherapist or something you enjoy doing on your own, like swimming laps in an outdoor pool in the morning, as recovery and strengthening of you vestibular ability. Do what you love to do.

The damage to your vestibular doesn't mean the end of good balance. You have the rest of your body receptors to help out with balance. Once you train and develop those receptors, they will help compensate your balance issues. After a vertigo attack, you will be able to feel stronger. More definite. In a shorter space of time.

The goal of V.R.T. (Vestibular Rehabilitation Therapy) is to retrain the brain to recognize and process signals from the vestibular system in coordination with information from vision and body. This often involves desensitizing the balance system to movements that provoke symptoms of imbalance.

Essentially, the brain copes with the disorientating signals coming from the inner ears by learning to rely more on the alternative signals coming from the eyes, ankles, legs, spine, neck and muscular system to maintain balance. Vestibular compensation can be successfully achieved even when the damage to the inner ear is permanent.

A qualified therapist will first give you a thorough evaluation. This includes observing your posture, balance, movement, and compensatory strategies you're already doing.

Using the result of this evaluation, the therapist will develop an individual treatment plan designed to include exercises that combine specific head and body movements with eye exercises and activities that you perform during therapy sessions and also do at home.

These exercises involve movements, of the eyes, the head, the upper body, and then the whole body under different visual situations (for example, with the eyes open or closed, or looking at steady objects or a moving ball), on different surfaces and in different environments. This is so helpful, as you and I have experienced the complexity of feelings that assault your sense of balance from our daily environment.

During sessions, the therapist will watch your eyes, while you move into different positions. In this way, the physiotherapist works with you to determine if certain positions of the head or visual environmental elements make the symptom worse. She or he will help you build up a tolerance for those elements that affect your balance.

As you can guess, some of the exercises and activities may at first cause an increase in symptoms, as body and brain attempt to sort out the new pattern of movements. A key factor is that the brain must sense the presence of imbalance to begin the process of vestibular compensation. So with time and consistent work, the signals from the eyes, body and vestibular system will start to co-ordinate again. This gives a greater sense of balance. Which is just what you need.

Activities and exercise are progressively increased in order to strengthen muscles and increase your tolerance for particular situations and conditions.

As you progress in your rehabilitation program to the more difficult vestibular exercises, you may experience dizziness when you do them. Don't be too worried about this. I know it's uncomfortable but it will improve, so that you don't experience that dizziness again. Also the exercises are slowly progressive and very controlled.

Here's where maintaining a positive approach pays off. Try not to think that an exercise will trigger an attack. That would be very unlikely. Don't see dizziness as a setback or a reason to stop. It just means that an imbalance between your left and right vestibular systems still exists and the exercises you are doing will help your brain detect the imbalance so it can gradually begin to accept it and compensate. However, when you are at home, don't push it so hard that you are sick or become exhausted. Please note that you should not attempt any of these exercises without first seeing a specialist or physiotherapist for a comprehensive assessment, advice and guidance. Your doctor can refer you.

Cawthorn-Cooksey Vestibular Exercises

Some physiotherapists work using a set pattern of exercises known as the Cawthorn–Cooksey exercises, named after the two people responsible for devising them. The aims of the Cawthorn-Cooksey exercises include relaxing the neck and shoulder muscles, training the eyes to move independently of the head, practicing good balance in everyday situations, practicing the head movements that cause dizziness (to help the development of vestibular compensation), improving general co-ordination, and encouraging natural spontaneous movement. You should be assessed for an individual exercise program to ensure you are doing the appropriate exercises for your specific issues. You will be given guidance on how many repetitions of each exercise to do and when to progress to the next set of exercises.

The exercises I mention below are not to be done without the supervision of a qualified therapist. It's just to give you an idea of what to expect. So don't try these at home just yet!

Sitting

Focus on your finger. Move your finger towards your face, starting from three feet away from your face. Follow your finger to one foot away from your face. Move your eyes slowly at first, then quickly).

Shrug and circle your shoulders. Bend forward and pick up objects from the ground. First from the left and then from the right. Side to side.

Standing

Move your eyes slowly at first, then quickly, up and down; from side to side. Then focus on your finger moving from three feet to one foot away from your face. Shrug and circle your shoulders. Change from a sitting to a standing position with your eyes open, and then closed. Throw a ball from hand to hand above eye level Throw a ball from hand to hand under the knees Change from a sitting to a standing position, turning around in-between.

Moving

Walk across the room with eyes open, then closed. Walk up and down a slope with eyes open, then closed. Walk up and down steps with eyes open, then closed (do this with supervision). Any game involving stooping, stretching and aiming is good to practice.

Vertigo Training In The Gym

You can manage vertigo symptoms by working out with weights. Controlled weight bearing exercise helps balance and strengthen your body equally on both sides. Even with vestibular damage, you can maintain your strength. People with vestibular damage often become body builders. Gym training or other challenging activities should always be done with a partner or personal trainer. Don't give up. With time, practice and commitment, you can do activities and sports that you were doing before you became ill and you may even discover new physical activities you hadn't even dreamed of doing. The idea is not to be limited by the fear of vertigo.

Identity

Goffman (1963) says "An individual carries a stigma if s/he is unable for any reason to fulfil society's stereotypic criteria for normality - if this deviation is obvious (e.g. physical deformity) the person is at once 'discredited'. Failings that are less obvious or may be concealed (e.g. vestibular problems) render the individual 'discreditable' in the sense that his/her identity is vulnerable. Whereas a discredited person must adopt a stigmatized identity - a discreditable individual may prefer the effort and risks attached to trying to 'pass' as normal to the frank stigma of admitting the attribute".

I can relate to what Goffman is saying here. I was one of the people who tried to pass as normal at work. I "acted" normal, as if I did not have anything wrong with me and dodged showing any symptoms. I didn't wish to have the stigma of admitting the symptoms because I felt my identity was extremely vulnerable. This identity issue is something you are going to need specialized help for. You must come to terms with it in a positive productive manner.

Vertigo is not just a physiological issue, it's also a psychological one. And this affects more than the moment of vertigo. It affects you on a daily basis. And it affects how you relate to others around you. Personally, I found that once I accepted that Meniere's was a permanent part of my life, I started to be able to work with and live with the symptoms.

Once I could accept the symptoms, I became more aware of how they were presented to me. I made changes to my lifestyle and attitude. And so the acceptance of the condition became, by default, part of the healing process. I was no longer battling and fighting myself and a condition. I accepted that it was up to me to make changes. So I did.

Feeling Bad Can Be Good

If you think you felt bad, well the good news is you're right! It's not your imagination.

'The Quality of Well-being Scale' is a scientific study. The quality of life factor for Meniere's sufferers has actually been tested and quantified by research. In this study, Meniere's is comparable to very ill adults with a life threatening illness such as Cancer or Aids. This was established when Meniere's sufferers were not even having acute episodes!

When having acute attacks, the Quality of Well-being for Meniere's sufferers is closer to a non-institutionalized Alzheimer's patient, an Aids victim, or a Cancer patient... six days before death. The research quantifies that Meniere's sufferers lose 43.9% from the optimum well-being position of normal people. They say Meniere's sufferers are the most severely impaired non-hospitalized patients studied so far. This score reflects major impairment in mobility, physical activity, social activity and clear thinking patterns. Meniere's patients are in the significantly depressed category. So if you think you are having difficulty with Meniere's it's not surprising.

This information puts experiences of depression, mobility, social difficulties and clear thinking into perspective.

As I have written in my other two books, the impact Meniere's has on your life will not always be understood by non-sufferers. I once read that a High Court Judge, a man of the highest social order, publicly stated on record that "Meniere's disease is a mere minor inconvenience." Now, don't you wish that was true! Until non-sufferers understand the impact of Meniere's disease, then sufferers are vulnerable on a physical, mental, emotional and financial level, because they may not receive the support necessary to cope. Worse, Meniere's sufferers have been financially disadvantaged and financially ruined by social systems and corporate institutions that should be supportive. Be aware that the opposite of empathy can be true.

People who suffer from the long term chronic condition of Meniere's lose touch with the possibilities of their potential. We often restrict our activities because we feel so bad. We won't extend ourselves and try new things. We find it difficult and become fearful of extending our limits. Fear makes cowards of us all. And we cease to discover what we may be capable of doing. Let's keep Meniere's disease in perspective. You have a disease that is NOT terminal! If you have Meniere's, you have the wonderful opportunity to work on your quality of life. And to have a life. You have more going for you than you think.

Life is on your side.

Go out and live it.

About Meniere Man

This bestselling author is an Australian born writer and an award-winning Executive Creative Director, and partner in a successful advertising agency. At the height of his business career and aged just forty-six, he suddenly became acutely ill. He was diagnosed with Meniere's disease. He began to lose all hope that he would fully recover his health. However the full impact of having Meniere's disease was to come later. He lost his health, his career and financial status as well.

It was his personal spirit and desire to get "back to normal" that turned his life around for the better. He decided that you can't put a limit on anything in life. Rather than letting Meniere's disease get in the way of life, he started to focus on what to do about getting over Meniere's disease.

With the advice on coping, healing, hope and recovery in his bestselling books, anyone reading the advice given, can make simple changes and find a way to get over Meniere's disease. As he went on to do.

These days life is different for the Author. He is a fit man who has no symptoms of Meniere's except for tinnitus and hearing loss in one ear. He does not take any medication. All the physical activities he enjoys these days require a high degree of balance: snowboarding, surfing, hiking, windsurfing, weightlifting, and riding a motorbike. All these things he started to do while suffering with Meniere's disease symptoms.

Meniere Man believes that if you want to experience a marked improvement in health you can't wait until you feel well to start. You must begin to improve your health immediately, even though you may not feel like it.

With a smile and a sense of humor, the

Author pens himself as Meniere Man, because Meniere's disease changed his life dramatically. Today he is an author of twelve books including four Bestsellers and two #1 Bestsellers. He is a writer, painter, designer and exhibiting artist. He is married to a writer. They have two children. He spends his time writing and painting. He loves the sea, cooking, traveling, nature and the company of family, friends and his beloved dog.

ADDITIONAL INFORMATION

If you enjoyed this book and you think it could be helpful to others, please leave a review for the book at amazon.com. amazon.co.uk or Goodreads. Thank you.

This book and other Meniere Man books are available worldwide from international booksellers and local bookstores including Amazon.com, Amazon.co.uk, Barnes & Noble Books. Available in paperback and Kindle.

MENIERE MAN BOOKS

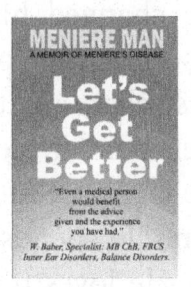

Let's Get Better
A Memoir of Meniere's Disease

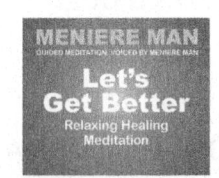

Let's Get Better CD
Relaxing & Healing Guided Meditation Voiced by Meniere Man

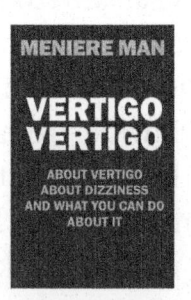

Vertigo Vertigo
About Vertigo About Dizziness and What You Can Do About it.

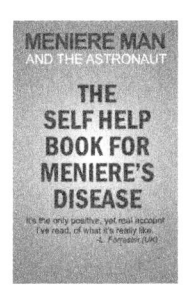

Meniere Man And The Astronaut
The Self Help Book for Meniere's Disease

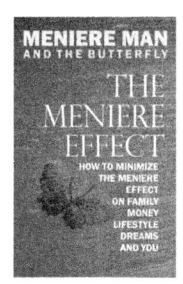

Meniere Man And The Butterfly
The Meniere Effect
How to Minimize the Effect of Meniere's on Family, Money, Lifestyle, Dreams and You.

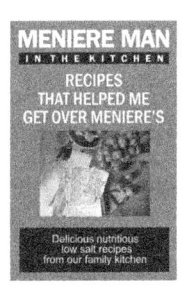

Meniere Man In The Kitchen.
Recipes That Helped Me Get Over Meniere's

MENIERE SUPPORT NETWORKS

Meniere's Society (UNITED KINGDOM)
www. menieres.org.uk
Meniere's Society Australia (AUSTRALIA)
info@menieres.org.au
The Meniere's Resource & Information Centre (AUSTRALIA)
www.menieres.org.au
Healthy Hearing & Balance Care (AUSTRALIA)
www.healthyhearing.com.au
Vestibular Disorders association (AUSTRALIA
)www.vestibular .org
The Dizziness and Balance Disorders Centre (AUSTRALIA)
www.dizzinessbalancedisorders.com
Meniere's Research Fund Inc (AUSTRALIA)
www.menieresresearch.org.au
Australian Psychological Society APS (AUSTRALIA)
www.psychology.org.au
Meniere's Disease Information Center (USA)
www.menieresinfo.com
Vestibular Disorders Association (USA)
www.vestibular.org
BC Balance and Dizziness Disorders Society (CANADA)
www.balanceand dizziness.org
Hearwell (NEW ZEALAND)
www.hearwell.co.nz
WebMD.
www.webmd.com
National Institute for Health
www.medlineplus.gov
Mindful Living Program
www.mindfullivingprograms.com
Center for Mindfulness
www. umassmed.edu.com